The Blessingway

Creating a beautiful Blessingway ceremony

Written by Veronika Sophia Robinson

Sept 2017

For Helen ♡

go create magic

♡ *Veronika* x x

The Blessingway

Creating a beautiful Blessingway ceremony
Written by Veronika Sophia Robinson

Published by Starflower Press
www.starflowerpress.com
July 3rd, 2012 ~ Full Moon in Capricorn
ISBN: 978-0-9560344-7-2
© Veronika Sophia Robinson

British Library Cataloguing in Publication Data.
A catalogue record for this book is available from the
British Library.

Also by the same author:

Fields of Lavender (poetry) 1991 ~ out of print.
The Compassionate Years ~ history of the Royal New Zealand Society for the Protection of Animals, RNZSPCA 1993
Peaceful Pregnancy CD, with Paul Robinson (The A Ffirm) 1995
Howl at the Moon (contributing poet), Wild Women Press 1999
The Drinks Are On Me: everything your mother never told you about breastfeeding (First edition published by Art of Change 2007) (Second edition by Starflower Press 2008)
Allattare Secondo Natura (Italian translation of *The Drinks Are On Me* 2009) published by Terra Nuova www.terranuovaedizioni.it
The Birthkeepers: reclaiming an ancient tradition (Starflower Press 2008)
Life Without School: the quiet revolution (Starflower Press 2010), co-authored by Paul, Bethany and Eliza Robinson
The Nurtured Family: ten threads of nurturing to weave through family life (Starflower Press 2011)
Natural Approaches to Healing Adrenal Fatigue (Starflower Press 2011)
Stretch Marks: selected articles from The Mother magazine 2002 – 2009, co-edited with Paul Robinson (Starflower Press)
The Mystic Cookfire: the sacred art of creating food for friends and family (more than 260 vegetarian recipes) (Starflower Press 2011)

With gratitude to my three ceremony mentors

Paul Robinson ~ my beloved ~ with love, respect and gratitude for your mesmerising ways with voice, gentle touch, and understanding of silence. As always: for being part of the greatest ceremonies and rituals of my life. You are my soul's love.

Rhonda Gola, Unity Celebrant, for encouraging and mentoring me as a marriage celebrant in 1995, and joining me in matrimony with my husband in a little chapel overlooking Green Bay, New Zealand, on December 29th, 1996. I thank you.

The late Jeannine Parvati Baker, my friend and colleague in conscious parenting, for initiating me into word-medicine, and supporting The Mother magazine so passionately from the start. You may be back with our Breathmaker, but I still feel your wisdom, wonder and wordcraft.

Dedicated to:
My Blessingway babies: ~ Bethany Angelika and Eliza Serena ~ now young women. You have truly blessed my way.

For the *amazing* women in my circle ~ the medicine wheel of my life ~ the ones who laugh, play, sip tea and coffee, write, pray, listen, phone, cry, care and love with and for me, from near and far. Go in peace.

Come Inside

'Birth is the most obvious expression of "what-is" that we can experience... For a conscious woman, childbirth is self-evidently holy. A spiritual midwife makes the full agreement to support the innate holiness of birth. It's as simple as this: anyone being with a woman giving birth, who worships, attends closely and invisibly, follows true, and opens hearts (as well as wombs), is a spiritual midwife.

A full spiritual midwife is a healer. She brings a commitment to maintain the wholeness of the birth experience, to keep it holy. She does no harm. In any effort to "save life", she will do no harm, create no extra karma.'

Jeannine Parvati Baker,
Psyche's Midwife, The Mother magazine

Navajo Blessingway Prayer

Hózhóogo naasháa doo
Shitsijí' hózhóogo naasháa doo
Shikéédéé hózhóogo naasháa doo
Shideigi hózhóogo naasháa doo
T'áá altso shinaagóó hózhóogo naasháa doo
Hózhó náhásdlíí'
Hózhó náhásdlíí'
Hózhó náhásdlíí'
Hózhó náhásdlíí'

In beauty may I walk.
All day long may I walk.
Through the returning seasons may I walk.
On the trail marked with pollen may I walk.
With grasshoppers about my feet may I walk.
With dew about my feet may I walk.
With beauty may I walk.
With beauty before me, may I walk.
With beauty behind me, may I walk.
With beauty above me, may I walk.
With beauty below me, may I walk.
With beauty all around me, may I walk.
In old age wandering on a trail of beauty, lively, may I walk.
In old age wandering on a trail of beauty, living again,
may I walk.
It is finished in beauty.
It is finished in beauty.

I was pregnant with my eldest daughter, Bethany, in 1995 when I first heard about the Navajo Blessingway ceremonies. I was living in New Zealand, and my American friend, Teresa, invited me to gift her with a bead to include in her Blessingway necklace. I was immediately intrigued, and couldn't wait to learn more. Little did I know then, how important Blessingway ceremonies would become in my own life, both as a mother and as a celebrant.

~ *Veronika Robinson, Summer Solstice, June 2012*

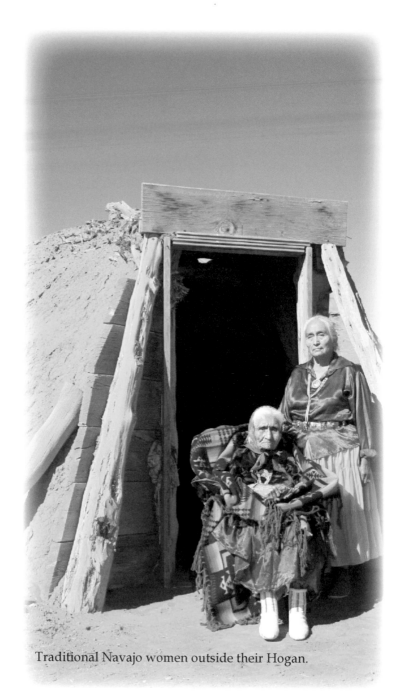

Traditional Navajo women outside their Hogan.

Hózhó jí
The Navajo Blessingway

'Our way of life is our religion, and our teaching. If we are relocated by force, we will die slowly. The people would not be in balance with Mother Earth and Sky Father and the spiritual people. In every way, here we are connected to the land. We belong here.' ~ Mary T Begay, Navajo Elder

Blessingway [Hózhó jí] ceremonies are performed for expectant mothers shortly before birth. The name of the rite, Hózhó jí, loosely translates as Blessingway, but this is word-medicine shorthand for well-being, success, harmony, beauty, perfection, orderliness, and ideal. In Navajo, this is for any stage of life and its transitions. What is common in all Blessingway ceremonies is the emphasis on the Hogan (home). In Navajo, the Hogan is considered a living object, and is loved and sustained by its inhabitants to maintain a harmonious family life.

The Navajo have many healing ceremonies based on chants and songs which Bless the Way of someone going through a rite of passage. These ceremonies are created to bring balance not only to the person involved, but to the world around them. Anthropologically, the Blessingway is one of the Navajo's six main ceremonies. The others are Gameways, Holyways, War ceremonials, Lifeways and Evilways.

A Blessingway is a positive ceremony, and traditionally lasted two nights. It was used to bring protection and blessings to a girl in menarche (first blood), or to a home, or to bring good fortune. It was also practised to ensure a healthy pregnancy and birth. This book is focused on the Blessingway ceremony as a rite of passage for a pregnant woman (and one who is adopting), and to bless her way into motherhood no matter how many or few children she already has. This is a sacred and spiritual occasion to the Navajo. Its use in Western society has been modified to suit the person involved and their own spiritual beliefs or lack thereof. The beauty of the Navajo traditions is that they don't see their connection to the Divine as isolated or separate from their daily activities. It's integrated into everything they do. Mother Earth, the plants, the animals, rivers, mountains, humans ~ they're all connected. It is through their prayers and ceremonies that the Navajo are able to understand and respect the balance and harmony between all living things and the Divine Creator.

The Navajo have a strong link to their land, and in particular have sacred sites where they offer up their prayers and ceremonies. The homelands of the Navajo are between the four sacred mountains: Blanca Peak in Colorado, Mount Taylor in New Mexico, the San Francisco Peaks in Arizona, and Hesperus Peak in Colorado. They understand that this will always remain their home, and that this is their sacred place on Earth.

Navajo families create a dwelling place (Hogan) which is built from four poles (posts) to represent the four sacred mountains. This packed-earth, dome-shaped home is built from bark, logs and dirt. Their home is part of the creation story: the earth floor is Mother Earth, and the round roof is a symbol of Father Sky. The family uses the Hogan for all religious ceremonies, and the more a place and space is used, the holier it becomes. This sacred use of space binds the Navajo to their land of birth.

'In our traditional tongue, there is no word for relocation.
To relocate is to move away and disappear.'
~ Pauline Whitesinger, Big Mountain Elder

When I planted my daughters' placentas under trees on the east coast of New Zealand's North Island, I knew it would symbolically tie them to the land of their birth, even though we would end up living on the other side of the world.

For the Navajo, when a baby is born the umbilical cord is buried close to the family Hogan. The cord has been nourished by the child's mother, and now, in the earth, is nurtured by Mother Earth ~ our spiritual mother. The placenta is buried under a tree, and the tree and child grow together through life. This bond is there for both of them. Navajo children grow up learning how to perform sacred ceremonies and rituals.

'Our offering places are sacred to us,
and the spiritual beings take care of us.
We know the land, the spiritual beings know us here.
If we leave our offering places, we will not be able to survive.'
~ Jack Hatathlie, Navajo Medicine Man

The Blessingway ceremony is considered the foundation of the Navajo life. It's based on the story of Changing Woman. She's the Earth through the changing seasons, and as such, is the major Navajo deity.

The story begins: First Woman and First Man came into this world in New Mexico, near Huerfano Mountain. First Man found a baby nearby, and in just four days the baby became Changing Woman. It's said that she created the original four Navajo clans. Her sons made the land safe for them to live. Her teachings include consecrating the Hogan for ceremonial use, as well as a girl's rite of passage through menarche. The Blessingway ceremony brings protection, peace, happiness and harmony. These rituals restore the body and spirit, and act curatively. In Navajo traditions, the ceremonies are performed by a Medicine Man. He uses plants, minerals, herbs and sand-paintings. The herbs and plants he gathers are from the local area, and are gathered for each ceremony at the time they're needed. They're not stored in any way. His job, when he sees a medicinal plant, is to tell it the name of a sick person. The plant is given offerings of prayers, pollen and songs. Given this in-depth consideration of the land and resources around them, it's easy to understand why the Navajo must remain on their sacred land.

The traditional Blessingway ceremony might appear simple, yet its ancient foundations are rich, beautiful and complicated. This two-day celebration begins with songs on the first night.

A ritual bath in yucca, with prayers and songs, is performed the next day. That evening, there's singing all night. Cornmeal and pollen are important in the ceremony. Dry paintings are created from vegetable materials such as flower petals, pollen and cornmeal.

When conducting your Blessingway ceremony, offer up a prayer of gratitude so that the guests become aware of your word-medicine. Be thankful for the blessings to all women and mothers, and say thank you to Changing Woman. "Let the Divine Mother be made manifest in this Blessingway."

The Celebrant

The celebrant is not the centre of attention in any ceremony. Her (his) job is to link the various elements and themes and lead the witnesses/congregation through the ceremony. Her role is to seamlessly join the beginning, middle and end, and to create a sacred space. She uses craft, pace and heart, and is there to 'hold' the energy and provide a safe container for what may emerge. This is a role of leadership, but ego needs to be left behind. A good leader leads without people realising they're following. Her job is to offer structure ~ like the spine ~ to the ceremony. It's important that she sets her intention, and that she asks herself "What does this ceremony mean?"

You don't need to be a professional celebrant to lead a Blessingway (or any other) ceremony. What you do need is a sense of calm, a professional attitude (even if you're doing this as a friend), and an awareness of human needs.

You'll need humility, dedication and a willingness to listen to inner guidance. When ceremony is an aspect of your daily life, you'll feel the sacred everywhere. If you're new to this, you can develop the craft. Sincerity is vital.

You'll need to have an understanding of the power of words as medicine, and the importance of symbols as a way of understanding and expressing human archetypes and myths.

When discussing with the mother-to-be the date and time of the ceremony, look beyond the diary. Connect with the season, and consider the different energies available: new Moon, full Moon, Solstice, Equinox. And the same goes for the time of day. Don't limit yourself to the numbers on a clock. Think about the Earth's rhythm: sunrise, sunset, noon, midnight.

Ideally, a Blessingway ceremony is held about the eighth Moon of pregnancy.

Other things to consider include the mother's beliefs; spiritual, religious or otherwise. What symbols, ideas, songs and readings does she wish to contribute? ·

When holding your script during the ceremony, keep it inside a hardback clothbound book. This is more professional than holding a piece of paper. Even if you're officiating as a best friend or sister, take care with your dress. Usually, celebrants avoid wearing sandals and having bare arms and feet. However, as a Blessingway celebrant, barefoot is fine if the venue encourages it, for example in someone's home or on the beach. Unlike other ceremonies, the celebrant will not stand in front of the guests, but be seated in the circle ~ opposite the guest of honour.

Avoid reading the ceremony script. Be familiar with the format, and make eye contact with everyone in the medicine wheel. Pronounce all of your consonants. The dropping of clear pronunciation is leading to the collapse of communication in our society. I encourage you to care enough about your spoken word and your audience, so that everyone understands what you're saying. If outdoors with a lot of people, always ask if everyone can hear you.

Even if the spoken words of the celebrant's contribution to the ceremony haven't been learnt, you should be at ease enough with what you're saying to be able to make it sound as if the thoughts are spontaneous and heartfelt. In actor's parlance, it means getting the words 'off the page'.

Practical tip: Use your role to encourage guests to use the toilet and their camera between activities, rather than during them.

Grounding

All celebrants should ground themselves before undergoing ceremonial duties. By doing so, you can bring down divine energies and connect with everyone in the circle. It allows you to be a conduit for Divine mind, and also protects you from potentially harmful energy.

To ground yourself, stand on some earth and breathe in deeply. Breathe out deeply. Allow yourself to really feel the earth beneath your feet, and keep breathing. Imagine that your breath is going through your feet, deep into Mother Earth. I like to imagine myself as a tree with my roots reaching deeper and deeper, secure, strong right down into the cold, dark, damp earth.

Our ancestresses lay beneath the ground of Mother Earth, holding us all. Let your roots travel down to these Ancient Mothers. Touch them.

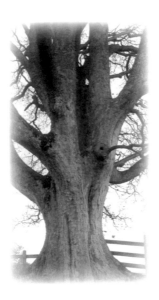

Go down even deeper, and feel the heat and heart of hot Mother Earth. If there's anything you need to release, perhaps a difficult journey to the ceremony or an unpaid bill on your mind, let it go. Give it to Mother Earth.

Now, let the love, power and beauty of our Earth Mother send her energy up to you right through your legs, your womb, your heart, your head. Keep breathing. Feel yourself expanded. There's so much energy inside you now. Let it expand outside of your body and out into the Universe.

Grounding yourself in this way allows you to become aware of everything around you. Your clarity will become precision-like.

With practice, grounding needn't take long ~ just a few conscious breaths. How do you know if you're grounded? Stand on one leg. If you can move the other leg without losing your balance, then you're grounded. Quick ways to ground include laughing, touching an animal or tree, carrying earth gems like tiger eye, obsidian or black tourmaline.

Creating Ceremony

Ritual and ceremony are intrinsic to human evolution; however, in modern culture our rituals for expansion, sacredness and blessing have been replaced by computer screens, TVs, mobile phones and isolated communities. We're bereft of meaning. And yet, our heart calls out for powerful rituals. This is the same for all of us whether we're religious, spiritual, agnostic or atheist.

When we move from one phase of our life to another ~ whether that's moving home, getting married or divorced, starting a new job or beginning/finishing university and so on ~ we instinctively want ways to mark such events. For many, this might end up being a drink at the pub, rather than what our soul is really calling for.

It is within ritual that we create significance around our transitions, and crafting sacred time and space into our days addresses a deep need, personally and culturally.

Wedding and funerals tend to be the key events of life where we stop what we're doing and attend, and yet there are so many other opportunities in life ~ some small, some large ~ which can be infused with sacred ceremony.

Ceremony offers healing, support, nourishment and protection.

At the heart of any ritual is the use of symbols, for they mirror an intention. They might seem insignificant but actually they're deeply powerful, because they use the left part of the brain ~ the dream side or inner child, and it allows us to heal in ways that mainstream medicine simply can't offer.

Consciously practised ritual enables us to enter a higher consciousness which changes the brain waves.

To successfully facilitate a ceremony requires having the awareness of noticing what is going on around you ~ a sixth sense about your environment. It's one thing to study ancient cultures, such as the Navajo, but it's another thing altogether to integrate their messages, and convey the meaning through our words and actions in a ceremony. If you're leading a ceremony, it is of benefit to everyone if you're in tune with what is happening around you ~ temperature, noise, group emotion, energy, smell, silence. This sensory awareness can be developed if you feel being in tune doesn't come naturally to you. Learning to pay deep attention to the little things around you will bring a deeper sense of awareness.

I find that the more time I spend in Nature, the more aware I become of the importance of finding silence in our lives. Ours is a 24/7 culture, which seeks to fill every second with noise of some sort. This generation of children is plugged in to TVs, computers, and mobile phones. Not many of them understand the healing energy and psychic importance of silence. As a celebrant, it's vital to not only ground yourself in Nature but to appreciate how rich this sensitivity to quiet is: personally, and to your practice of creating meaningful ceremony. When facilitating a ceremony, learning to use silence between your words, and your sentences, helps to give you gravitas, and draws the audience in to your words so they can truly listen.

Inviting your guests to be conscious of the silence, and to allow silence, is beneficial too.

The ceremony of a Blessingway is a way of getting to know the mother, and nourishing her onward journey. It's a gift to her, and to the participants, which far outstrips the material gifts of modern life.

The beauty of the Blessingway ceremony is that it spans the generations, and is a potent vision quest not only for the mother-to-be, but her community and family, as they prepare for the birth of new life. The rituals allow each person involved to access different parts of themselves. As witnesses to the mother, we each affirm that birth (or adoption) will be beautiful, peaceful and natural.

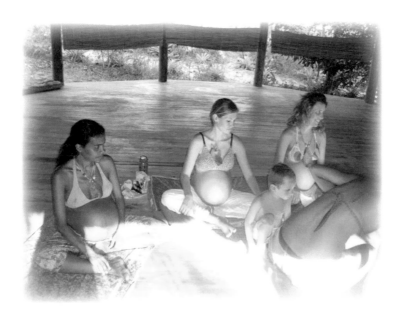

A Blessingway ceremony in Brazil.

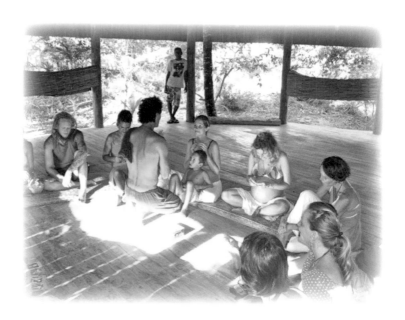

Many people will feel their fears about birth (or more accurately, death) come to the surface. As a Blessingway celebrant, it's important to address these fears.

The ceremony is an opportunity to talk about the mother's dream life, if she so wishes. Who has she met upon the road of her dreams? What are her fears? How can we help her let them go? What roadblocks stand between her and her baby's natural birth?

As I explored in my book, *The Birthkeepers: reclaiming an ancient tradition*, death is often the greatest fear women have in relation to birth. Birth and death are part of the same story, and to deny the possibility that one might die in birth is not helpful to anyone. A shamanic approach to this is to accept the *possibility* of death, and to explore it as a rite of passage. We can look at what death means in other cultures, and we can also explore the symbolism of death: the closing of a door, and walking through a new one. A labyrinth is a wonderful healing tool for letting go of such fears. (see page 61)

We learn that birth is not just physical, but spiritual, too. The mother-to-be may discover that this is a rare opportunity in her life to unify mind, body and soul. Great healing occurs when we face our fears. The key to accepting the possibility of death is surrender ~ and this is true regardless of where, when and how we birth. Surrendering to your body's power, and the co-creative dance with your baby, is a shamanic peak experience.

A sacred ceremony bridges the link between our human existence and our divine origins. We remember we're of both Heaven and Earth. Ceremony is about intention, and can be considered as prayer in action.

We don't need to wait for crises in our lives before yearning for contact with our spiritual source ~ we can access it any time. The use of items from our material world, for example: water, fire, earth, air ~ feathers, flowers, crystals, etc., is important in ceremony. I like to create an altar, and in doing so, set forth my intention for the ceremony. Regardless of the intention, deep, conscious breathing is vital for experiencing the Divine, and will ensure that the ceremony you create is in alignment with your deepest intentions.

The mother-to-be can be encouraged to see her Blessingway ceremony as the blueprint for her baby's birth. There are the opening rituals which symbolise labour, and the gifts from her guests are like giving birth. How does she receive them? Is she open? Is she grateful? Is she happy?

The closing of the circle with prayers and music is like the delivery of the placenta. If you're highly sensitive and aware, you'll be able to 'read' how the woman 'gives birth' in her ceremony, and share the vision you saw.

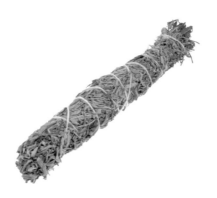

Sage stick for smudging.

Sacred Space

The choice of site for the Blessingway ceremony should be decided by the mother-to-be, and it's wise for her to consider where she feels most empowered, and filled with joy and happiness. For some women, this will be in their own home, where they'll give birth; for others, it will be in their garden, a field or the woods.

As the celebrant, create your circle. Use stones, cornmeal, seashells, driftwood, sticks, pine cones. Wherever the location, create a peaceful and relaxing atmosphere. Use candles, soft lighting (if indoors), relaxing music, fabric, saris and cushions.

Your role as celebrant will be to remind guests to leave behind negative, fearful stories and comments. It goes without saying: *mobile phones should be turned off.* Remind your guests to turn them off. If indoors, put the phone on mute, and turn the answering machine down. Put a note on the front door: *Do Not Disturb.*

Create an altar in the centre with objects from your medicine bag or the mother's special items. Ideally, you will have had meetings before the ceremony. If she has left the altar for you to prepare, then create one incorporating her beliefs.

You can place drawings of the Goddesses, or statues of deities such as Buddha, Jesus Christ, Mother Mary, Kali, Krishna, Shiva, etc. Draw in the four directions, and place a symbol for each element. Spring water; crystal for earth; candle for fire; feather or incense for air. Consider the fifth element: the etheric world, and maybe include a mandala.

My medicine bag contains: velvet cloth, beeswax candles, owl feathers, an amethyst and other gemstones, hemp red thread, a bell, sage, Nag champa incense, a Buddha statue, silver-birch sticks.

The Blessingway is a celebration to honour, empower and nurture the mother-to-be as well as the new life she's carrying. The sacred space you're creating needs to be gentle, intimate, peaceful, safe and comfortable. As a celebrant, your ceremony will aim to unify the energy of all in attendance.

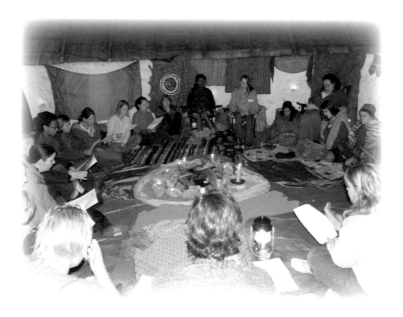

Singing Blessingway songs around the medicine wheel inside the roundhouse at The Mother magazine family camp.

The Altar

You don't have to be spiritual or religious to have a Blessingway ceremony held for you, or to officiate a ceremony. I do feel, though, it's best if the person chosen for the role of celebrant has a great affinity with Nature, through all the seasons, and loves being outdoors, as well as having an awareness of her six senses.

Most celebrants have an altar or several altars in their home or garden. If you're new to ceremony, an altar is a sacred space where we go to connect with the Divine.

An altar is created in a place that is away from the busyness of our day-to-day lives. The size doesn't matter. It can be a whole room devoted to your worshipping, or the size of a book. It is a place where we go to reflect on our growth: spiritual and personal.

Throughout history, humans in all cultures have used an altar in their worship. It aligns us with our deep need to connect with a power greater than us. Our soul needs as much nurturing as our body, and an altar invites us to pause and be. Worship is private, and yet, in group ceremony it is right that we have a group altar, as this is a shared worship. It's a focal point for our collective transformation ~ spiritually, emotionally, physically and mentally. The balance we all seek is found in the relation-ship we have with the Universal Power. Spiritual health is as vital to our well-being as the health of our other bodies ~ physical, emotional and mental.

At home, you may have your altar in the garden, on a bookshelf, window ledge, a corner of the room. It's kept free from anything not related to worship, and is tended to each day. Flowers are kept fresh, and the space dusted or cleaned.

Items which find their way to the altar should be symbolic of your sacred connection to the Universe. They can represent your beliefs, your family, your relationship to Nature. As with ceremony, the power of intention is the foundation of creating an altar. Including Nature in her various forms is especially potent: feathers, stones, flowers, plants, herbs, berries, seeds, flower essences, crystals and gems. Animal statues can represent totem animals, and may remind you of the strength or wisdom you're seeking.

Incense from Tibetan monasteries is almost always used on altars. The scent diffuses energies in the room. My favourites are Maroma and Nag Champa. As you breathe in the scent, it sends a message to your mind that worship is beginning. Your vibration matches your intention. Ensure you use 100% genuine incense.

The altar will contain at least one candle, to announce your intention.

A Blessingway altar is ideally created by the mother-to-be or created from symbols she's chosen and given to you. As a celebrant, you can give guidance on their purpose, and what she might like to include, and why: a beeswax candle, sage, fertility symbols, blessing beads, feathers, a statue or photo of chosen deity, flowers which have fallen naturally, a bowl of water, crystals, a bell to change the energy before and after the ceremony, incense, fruits and seeds to represent fertility and life.

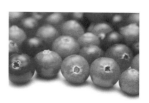

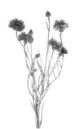

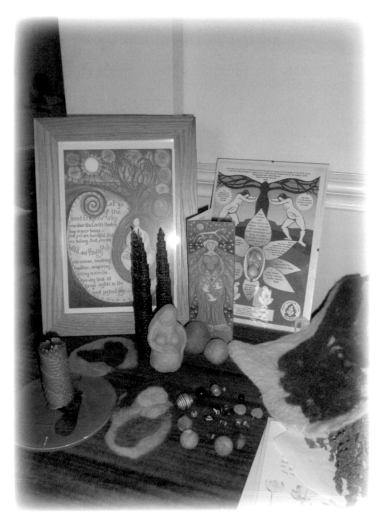

Karen's Blessingway altar.

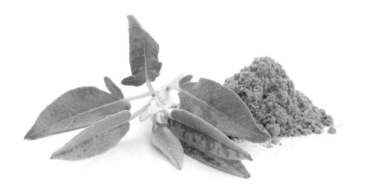

The Native American Indians believe sage is one of Earth's oldest plants, and consider it important in spiritual cleansing. Try to have some ~ fresh or dried ~ on the altar, even if you're not sage smudging.

Look to include the four elements: fire ~ candle; water ~ shell or dish of spring water; air ~ feather, incense; earth ~ crystal or dirt.

When seeking gifts from Nature for the altar, ask permission from the spirits of the land or plant. Ask that you may receive, rather than take.

Lay a velvet or similar cloth on top of the surface before laying down the symbols. Where possible, have the altar in the centre of the circle. When your altar is created, give thanks.

The Four Directions

At the beginning of the ceremony, invoke the spirits of the four directions. Ideally, do this out loud and include it in your ceremony script. If this is something the mother isn't comfortable with, then you can do this silently before you start.

"I call to the spirit of the East."
"I call to the spirit of the South."
"I call to the spirit of the West."
"I call to the spirit of the North."

According to the Native American Medicine Wheel, we find the following symbols for each direction:

EAST ~ inspiration, air, birth, yellow, Spring, activity, waxing Moon, owl (eagle), dawn, mind.

SOUTH ~ intuition, water, nurturing, Summer, childhood, dolphin, blue, noon, full Moon, emotions.

WEST ~ transformation, fire, Autumn, red, adult, snake (phoenix), sunset, spirit/soul, experimenting, waning Moon.

NORTH ~ introspection, earth, Winter, black/white, elder, new Moon, consolidation, turtle (bear), body, midnight.

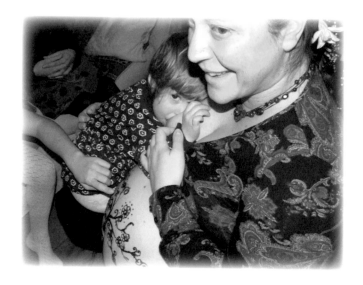

Johanneka breastfeeding during her mum's henna painting.

The Medicine Wheel

It's up to the mother to decide if she wants her ceremony to be a women-only Blessingway, or if men (fathers,
brothers, sons, grandfathers) are welcome. She might
choose to have adults only, and no children. There are no
hard-and-fast rules. The choice of guests, however, will
change the nature of the ceremony, but there's no right or
wrong, and deep healing can happen for any guest in the
medicine wheel.

Increasingly, women want their partners at the ceremony, because it represents his place as her lover and in
family life. As Jeannine Parvati Baker suggested, creating
gentle birth allows the masculine energies on this Earth to
be healed. Consider a dual-gender Blessingway ceremony
as a step towards a more harmonious culture.

As a celebrant, you'll simply include the father
alongside the mother in your rituals. They sit, side by
side, in the North.

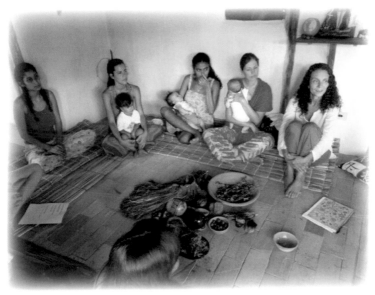

Around the Medicine Wheel in Brazil.

Jamie, pregnant with Kobra.

When inviting guests, let them know they can consciously prepare for the ceremony by bathing themselves and wearing ceremonial clothing. That is, dressing in clothes to mark the special occasion rather than wearing the jeans they've been in all week.

I've facilitated ceremonies where toddlers are in attendance. Ideally, the circle becomes the parent, so that any roving child is guided by whoever is closest, rather than the parent having to move about the circle all the time. *A practical tip:* keep the altar and all candles out of reach of toddlers.

One thing to be mindful of: mobile (young) children often end up becoming the centre of attention, and the focus shifts to them rather than the mother-to-be. This ceremony could be one of the few times the mother gets to have time for her, and her alone, so where possible this should be honoured. I feel that in-arms breastfed babies are naturally at home in the circle and don't detract from the ceremony. If he's unsettled, then the baby's mother should discreetly move out of the circle until he's content.

A Blessingway, ideally, wouldn't have more than about 12 to 15 guests, and probably no fewer than about five. I have, however, facilitated Blessingways with about thirty guests (there were three pregnant women being blessed in the ceremony). The intention should be for an intimate ceremony, and guests should only be invited if they truly mean something to the mother, rather than being invited out of obligation.

When we witness an event, we're neurally experiencing it, so in a Blessingway ceremony the guests of the medicine wheel are as much a part of the Blessingway transformation as the mother-to-be.

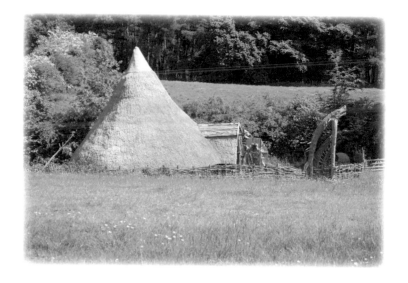

Limetree Farm ~ home of The Mother magazine family camps. The stone circle and the roundhouse make beautiful circles within which to hold ceremonies.

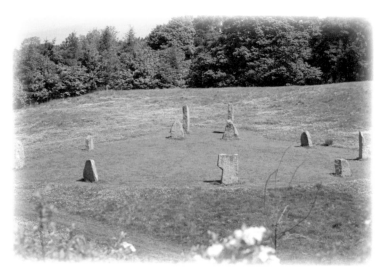

Casting the Circle

As a celebrant, you'll need to invite everyone into the circle. If guests have been gathering and chatting beforehand, your role is to gently call their attention to the fact the ceremony will soon begin. Invite them to come into the circle, and suggest that they might like to focus on their breathing for a few minutes: encouraging them to breathe deeply, conscious of the inhale and exhale.

There are many ways to open the circle. You might, for example, choose a talking stick, flower, stone, ball of red thread or pine cone where each person takes it and says their name, or a greeting. The energy you're trying to create will ensure that each participant is fully present. In some cases, it's appropriate to acknowledge that they've travelled from some distance and to use these few moments to let go of their journey, or whatever has happened in the day, so that they can be fully present to witness the ceremony.

I ask for the circle to be open, and on behalf of the person for whom the ceremony is intended, thank everyone for being there, and express my honour and privilege at being part of such a ceremony.

One thing to consider is whether you want the mother in the circle before you begin, or if you'd like to invite her in after everyone has settled into their place in the medicine wheel. Ideally, I like to have the altar prepared, the circle created, candles lit around the circle, and guests seated...and then I invite the mother in before the sage-smudging begins. I invite her in with the sound of my bell ringing three times. This announces the start of the ceremony. The look on a mother's face when she walks into a dark room lit by candles, and transformed with red fabrics, cushions and loving faces, is priceless.

To clear the space where your ceremony is held, it's a good idea to move the energy by introducing something different. For example, you can brush the air, floor, walls

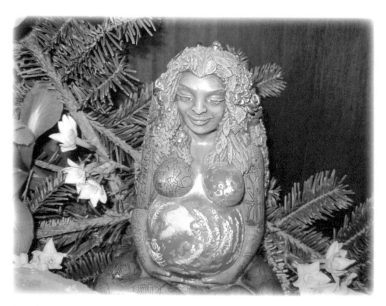

Earth Mother on Kathryn's Blessingway altar.

with sage, or spritz the air with essential oils of lavender or lemon myrtle. You could have a bowl of spring water over which you've given your blessings in meditation, and then ask guests to pass it around the circle. They could place their fingers in it, then pass it to the next person. When everyone has had a turn, you can place the bowl on the altar. Some celebrants prefer to use salt, and sprinkle that around the space. You might like to brush guests with a feather.

Find an element that you and the mother are comfortable with, and integrate this into the opening of your ceremony. If you're performing the ceremony in someone's living room, ask permission to rearrange the furniture a bit. This not only makes more space, it helps to change the energy.

The origins of the Navajo Blessingway ceremony reveal that they would 'smudge' the Hogan with a bundle of dried sage. The sage is lit, and the flame dies down slowly. This cleansing prepares the home for childbirth. The Navajo believe that it purifies the woman's soul, and blesses her and her baby for birth.

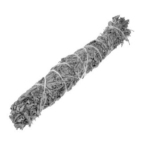

The witnesses at the ceremony are also smudged. This can be done with sage or incense. A feather or branch of cedar or lavender can also be used by the celebrant as she walks around the medicine wheel ensuring everyone in the circle is cleansed.

The mother-to-be sits in the North of the circle, and is made a special seat with cushions or pillows, and with a sense of it being like a royal throne. If possible, have her seat raised in exaltation so that she's higher than her witnesses. If her midwife or doula is in attendance, they'll sit in the West (unless they've taken on the role of celebrant, in which case they should sit opposite).

Your intention when casting the circle is to bring fresh energy and a sense of newness. This is the time in the ceremony when I remind guests that what we're participating in is as old as the Navajo Indians, and as young as the baby here in utero. Together we affirm the pregnant woman will have a beautiful, ecstatic birth experience. That is our wish. This is the moment to remind women that they're sacred. They're goddesses. They are: *Mother Earth made manifest.*

It's very important as a celebrant to lift your words off the page so each single one has meaning and resonance. Each sentence of your ceremony is rich word-medicine capable of great healing. Don't read your script. Be familiar with it, and by all means refer to it. You don't need to know it word for word, but you do need to let the words live and breathe. Let them rise from the page and out to those present. Sound all of your consonants, and ensure that your voice is heard by everyone.

We have formed in a circle, and singing the Blessingway song *Circle Surrounding* raises the energy and lifts everyone to a new place. They let go of wherever they've come from, and are now present and able to be witnesses to the pregnant woman's rite of passage.

Circle Surrounding
There's a circle surrounding the circle we are in
(three times)
The Angels, Beings of Light
Calling in the Angels, to be by our side
Knowing, when we call them
Their light is here to guide our way
Their light is here to guide.
© The Blessingway CD, Copperwoman

Every venue or location brings with it its own energy. I've officiated many types of ceremonies in a variety of locations, such as open fields by woodland, an Ironage roundhouse replica, yurts, homes, Maori marae, a stone circle, botanical gardens, by an ancient spring, a river, and bushland.

Wherever the ceremony is held, be mindful that you still need to create a circle. If the venue of choice is a home, such as the living room, be conscious about what might take the energy away. For example, cover the television with a pretty cloth. Tidy up toys or newspapers if the mother hasn't already done so. Clean and clear the space. If the Blessingway is during the day, you might like to close the curtains and light the room with candles. Use your senses when creating the ceremony atmosphere: sight, sound, smell, touch.

Yurts and bell tents are wonderful for ceremonies like this because they cast a circle energetically before you even add your symbols. They 'hold' the medicine wheel.

If your event is outdoors, such as a garden, park, beach, field or woodland, use the elements of your environment to help you cast the circle. For example, sea shells, seaweed, driftwood, pine cones, stones, branches or fallen flowers. You'll need to take into account issues such as privacy, roadside noise, weather conditions, ease of access for guests (especially if heavily pregnant), and to remember every item you'll need for the Blessingway ceremony.

Consider how you will use cushions, cloths, candles, incense, altar table and symbols, fabrics for wall hangings, and music during the Blessingway.

Silence

When a celebrant practises silence in her (his) life, it will permeate the way s/he officiates sacred ceremonies. It is within the sound of silence that the whole Universe exists. There are many names for this, such as God, Goddess, All that is, Truth, Love, I Am, Holy Spirit. This is the 'peace that passeth all understanding'. And yet, though it is a mystery we may not fully appreciate or understand, it exists within us, and when we can learn to recognise it, we shall hear the holy sounds of the Universe. With silence comes a respect for simplicity, and here is the key element of what a celebrant brings to her ceremonial work. She understands what it is to revere, and this is inherent in her ceremonies ~ regardless of the beliefs of those for whom she is the celebrant.

Silence has always played an important part in my life, and I see how vital it is to integrate this into celebrancy work. In ceremony, it allows friends and family to be given the space and time to connect with their inner world, as well as strengthening and deepening their relationship to the environment they're in.

Many people will be familiar with silent moments during a funeral, but it's just as powerful in Blessingways and other ceremonies, too. Incorporating it into the beginning of the ceremony, while you wait for the mother-to-be to enter the circle, will set the intention that this is a ceremony with purpose and power.

For some people, silence is uncomfortable and they may be used to filling every waking moment of their lives with noise. This is okay. You're offering them the opportunity to enjoy the beauty around them, and be fully present. It evokes a sense of something greater than one's self. Depending on the size of the group you're working with, you might have guests who giggle or whisper from nervousness. You can minimise this by being clear at the outset about how long the silence will last, and what your cue will be to bring it to an end. I will often offer up something for them to place their focus on ~ such as a candle, flower, or the mother-to-be, so that they can channel their intention.

As already mentioned, your role as celebrant is to lift your 'script' off the page. It should be inherent within your delivery that moments of silence fall appropriately, like traffic lights, where the written word has punctuation. Conscious approaches to the spoken word help to eliminate unnecessary word fillers like 'um', 'er', 'you know'.

The silence between the words is a gift to the guests around the medicine wheel ~ because they also have to slow down and digest what is being shared. They become present, not only to the external environment, but to their inner one, too.

Where do you use these silences? They're best placed just before or just after something you really wish to emphasise. Silences also ensure that your guests stay tuned. If you gabble through the ceremony, they'll tune out. Silence brings people to attention, and keeps them focused.

Offer silence in places where it would fall naturally, and keep your tone conversational rather than forced. If you need to, record yourself speaking the ceremony so you can get a sense of what the guests will hear.

I've felt very powerful emotion emanating from people when they're given the space for silence, and I can really feel their love for the mother-to-be, and from the community surrounding her.

As a celebrant, you can also use the power of silence before you begin the ceremony by grounding yourself, smiling, and making eye contact around the medicine wheel. This is welcoming to all concerned.

Ancient Mother

Ancient mother, I hear you calling
Ancient mother, I hear your song
Ancient mother, I hear your laughter
Ancient mother, I taste your tears
O la ma ma wa ha su kay la
O la ma ma wa ha su om
O la ma ma ka way ha ha ha ha
O la ma ma ta te ka kay
© Blessingway songs CD, by Copperwoman

Calling in the Ancient Mothers

Near the beginning, invoke the energy of our fore-mothers. In the circle, I ask the energy of the angels to be with us, including everyone's guardian angel, the angel of the land we're on, and any other supportive energies of the non-physical world. Even when a mother isn't open to invisible energies, she's generally receptive to the idea of our ancient mothers. We call upon our mothers, grandmothers and great-grandmothers throughout time to be with us during this sacred rite of passage, and we celebrate the long line of women who gave birth to us. We affirm our meeting in this sacred space as witnesses on our friend's journey into motherhood. The celebrant leads the call for the ancient mothers, and then encourages each woman in the circle (clockwise) to share their maternal ancestry: *my name is Veronika, and I'm the daughter of Angelikah, granddaughter of Liselotte and Minna Marie.*

Some women will be deeply moved by putting this into words and speaking it out loud. It may be the first time in their lives that they've verbalised their maternal lineage. Some women may be estranged from their mother; others may have deceased mothers; and others may have been adopted. If they're moved to tears, offer a tissue. Refrain from trying to 'fix' someone's sadness, overwhelm, gratitude or grief. Simply let them have their experience. Don't try and control their emotions. Let them flow freely.

If they can't find the words, give them a few moments and then say *'(person's name), we'll come back to you when you're ready. Take your time'.*

Don't panic. This is a healing ceremony, and emotions can and do arise. Your role as a celebrant is to hold the space. People won't feel safe to express their emotions if you lose your centre. When the ancient mothers have been called in, this is the right place to sing the Blessing-way song: Ancient Mother.

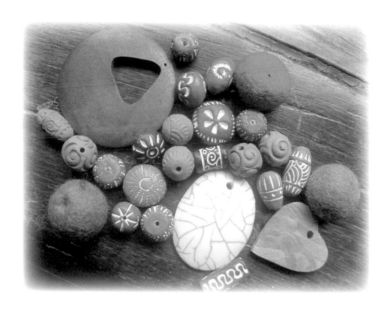

Blessingway beads (above) made from natural products.
Below: Kathryn's Blessingway beads.

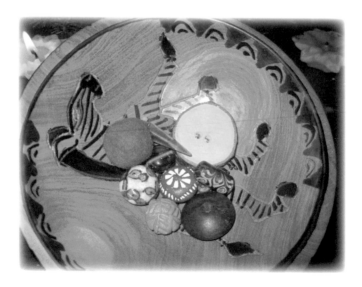

Ceremonial Gifts

In Blessingway ceremonies, the guests honour the mother-to-be with gifts, but it should be recognised that in this ceremony we're all learning to give birth to ourselves. This is a conscious exploration of the feminine (even for men, if they're included in the ceremony).

Through giving birth, we're expressing our sacred sexuality. It is an act of worship we share with the Goddess as well as our community.

There are many ways to add to the modern-day Western version of the Blessingway ceremony that aren't part of the Navajo tradition. Don't try and include all of them in the ceremony, as it will make it too long. Find two or three that most resonate with the mother-to-be.

As a celebrant, especially if you're also the midwife or doula, consider the way the mother-to-be receives her gifts. How open and grateful is she? This is symbolic of how she will open to labour and birth. Let your role, as celebrant, be to breathe deeply, and be aware of how the mother is breathing. It might be useful to gently suggest that this is mirroring the 'giving birth' part of her baby's journey Earthside.

The intention we set, as celebrants, when beginning a ceremony, is held by the participants in the medicine wheel. Doing so creates a group consciousness, and this raises the energy because everyone knows and can feel the goal. This is incredibly powerful, and builds up to a climax, just as in lovemaking. It releases the power for the benefit of all.

Every act and every symbol which is part of the Blessingway will raise the energy, whether it's the bead ceremony, brushing the pregnant woman's hair, prayer, bellydancing, chanting, singing, silence, clapping, henna, or playing an instrument. They all bring conscious intention to the sacredness of the ceremony.

Beads

The beading ceremony has become the most included one in the modern Blessingway. The mother-to-be or the celebrant sends an invitation to special guests for a bead. When they attend the ceremony, they'll hand over their chosen bead and share why that bead was special and 'called' to them. They may also use this opportunity to express their deepest wishes for the mother, and their hopes for her birth.

One by one, the guests will place their bead directly into the mother's hands, or a bowl, and as they go around the circle they'll share their bead story and message.

Traditionally, the birthing woman would thread the beads onto string while she was in labour, thereby drawing on the energy of all the women in her community.

I chose to thread my beads in labour, but some women choose to thread them during the ceremony or at another time which suits them.

I love the stories associated with my daughters' Blessingway beads. Bethany's beads contain a guitar plectrum so she'll foster a love of music. She's now almost an adult, and not only plays guitar but also violin, piano and flute, and is set on her path as a composer.

One of the beads was from a lovely Maori friend. Bethany had never met her nor had she seen a photo of her. When Bethany was about fifteen, she described what my friend looked like simply from holding the bead she'd given.

Eliza's beads have two dolphins made from tiger's eye. They were each given by twins, but here's the incredible thing: neither of them knew what bead the other one had brought! She also has beads that were from her great grandmother Eliza's jewellery (we didn't know that she was going to be called Eliza at this point), as well as handmade paper mâché beads from her relatives on the other side of the world. I love that these women in the family,

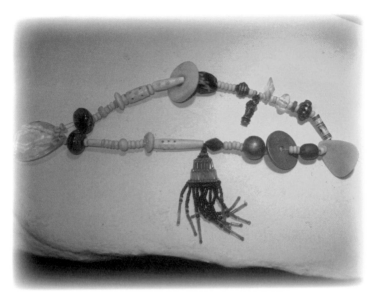

Bethany's Blessingway necklace with beads from around the world.

whom we'd never met, gathered together to be part of this unfamiliar ritual, to make beads by hand. It was truly beautiful, and when we met just over a year later, I felt the love and energy they'd already shared.

The most aesthetically pleasing beads are made from natural materials, such as wood, glass or felt. If it feels appropriate, include this suggestion in your invitations. Ask the guests to avoid plastic, if possible, as it's made from petrochemicals, and not conducive to caring for our Mother Earth.

Beads can be round, square or flat. Just ensure they have a hole for threading.

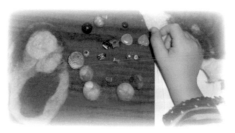

Karen's Blessingway beads.

Traditionally, the birthing woman would thread the beads onto string while she was in labour, thereby drawing on the energy of all the women in her community.

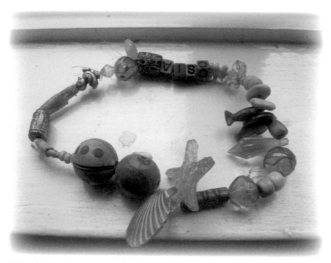

Eliza's Blessingway beads.

Blessingway Box

Use a box made from natural products such as willow or bamboo, and place a few items inside to remember the pregnancy. The mother-to-be can add to this later on. Items which might be included: raspberry-leaf tea; a picture of a Goddess; affirmations for an easy, ecstatic birth; a Blessingway necklace; flowers from her floral crown; a beeswax candle; a photo of her pregnancy; a Blessingway/birth phone tree.

Prayer Flags

This is a creative addition to any Blessingway ceremony. Invite the guests to bring a small, blank piece of fabric about 15x25cm, or provide the fabric and art items such as fabric pens, scissors, needles, thread, cookie-cutter shapes. Invite each guest to write a message or symbol. E.g. *Birth is safe. My body knows how to give birth.*

Symbols such as a sunflower about 10cm wide (to match a fully dilated cervix) or waves (to show labour) are perfect.

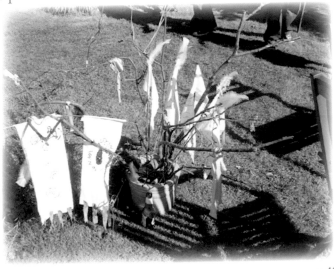

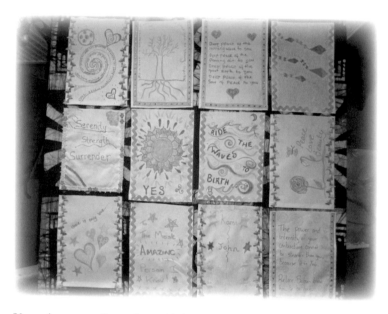

Karen's prayer flags: beautiful, colourful and positive!

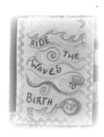

How to Make Blessingway Prayer Flags

1. Cut pieces of fabric to approximately 15 x 25cm.
A simple fabric like calico works well.

2. At the top of each piece, fold it down about a couple
of centimetres, and stitch along the top to make a sleeve
through which you can draw string.

3. Decorate the flags in any way that feels good: you can
appliqué, stitch, embroider, paint, stencil, glue on symbols, or write words such as: easy birth, open, love, joy,
peace.

4. When the flags are dry/ready, thread them with cord.
They can be hung outside between trees, or in the birthing
room, as a visual affirmation.

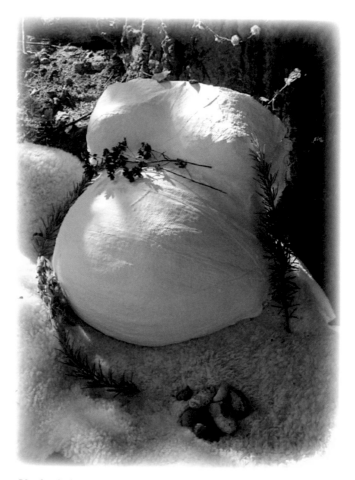

Keeley's bellycast from her pregnancy with Tansy.

Bellycast

The bellycast of a pregnant woman is as unique as her fingerprint. No two women have the same-sized-and-shaped breasts and belly. The mask is a three-dimensional plaster-of-Paris casting of her belly (and breasts, thighs, if desired). When the plaster has dried, the woman (and her community, if she wishes) can paint and decorate it. Some women prefer to leave their cast unadorned.

This way of capturing the last month of pregnancy can be used as a wall hanging, or turned upside down for a fruit bowl. Some women line it with cloth, and place their new baby inside for a photo, and other women have it framed as a 3D picture.

You can purchase a bellycast kit or buy the supplies yourself from a chemist.

How to make a belly cast

Before commencing any casting, place a large cloth on the floor ~ the sort that painters use is good.

The casting takes about twenty minutes, so it's generally a good idea for the mother-to-be to sit. She'll need to wait another ten minutes for it to dry. Place a cloth on her chair, too.

You'll need at least a couple of rolls of plaster bandage. Cut these into 15cm strips. You'll need a large bowl. Fill it with very warm water.

The mother will need to be unclothed on the part of her body being cast, for example: belly, breasts, thighs, depending on her choice. Some women keep their bra on because they feel modest. Always check in and see what she's comfortable with. Place plastic film over her bra.

Many people use petroleum jelly on the area of the skin to be cast. **Don't!** It's a derivative from the petroleum industry (hence the name) and is toxic. Use coconut or olive oil.

Belly Painting

Some women paint their bellies, not with henna, but eco-friendly body paints. There's no limit to the style of artwork which can be created on the canvas of a pregnant mother's belly.

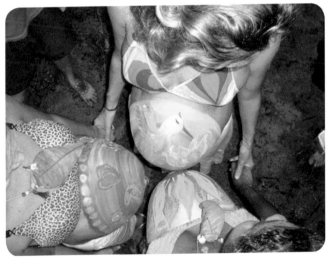

Beautiful bellies painted during a Brazilian Blessing-way ceremony.

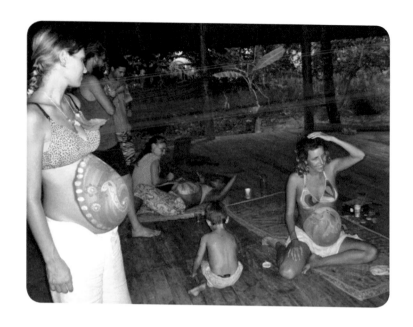

The Blessing Bowl

The blessing bowl can be made from felt, wood or other natural materials. Here, the guests in the medicine wheel place a blessing for the mother to have on her birth altar.

Blessings come in the form of affirmations, such as:

Your body is beautiful.
You are made to give birth easily.
Your body knows how to open.
Birth is pleasurable.
Your baby knows how to be born.
It is safe to give birth.

Journal

Give the mother a beautiful journal which she can write in or collate pictures and photos. During the Blessingway ceremony, each guest can include something to help the mother remember the power of her community, and be inspired for her journey ahead. Items might include: a recipe, poem, wish, prayer, parenting tip. Ask guests ahead of time for their contribution.

Photo Frame

Purchase or make a large wooden frame, and then invite each guest to add a symbol of fertility, which can be glued to the frame. For example, a shell or an egg. A photo of the mother during the Blessingway ceremony can be added to the frame later on.

Treasure Mapping

You will need:
Scissors, glue, colourful magazines
A large sheet of cardboard

Cut out positive words and photos to depict the birthing journey. Everyone can search for these treasures, and the mother can stick her favourite ones on the cardboard. She can then hang this in her birthing room.

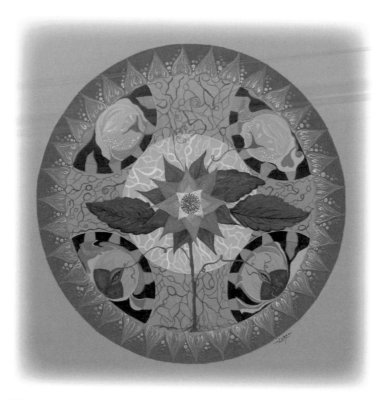

This mandala is called *Florecer*, which translates as Blossoming, and was created in 2008 by artist Lorena Leonardis Schernberg
www.SaludArte.ch, www.facebook.com/LoresMandalas

Lorena selected this mandala for the book because a blossoming flower is like the birth of a new person.

Mandala

The Cosmos can be seen in a mandala, which is a Sanskrit word to represent an energy circle. This is believed to bring protection. The elements of psychology, healing and sacred geometry are inherent in the consciousness of 'meditative-mandala making'.

The mandala maker tends to look towards the centre, and is deeply relaxed during their creation of art in the circle. Great biochemical changes occur in the brain because both hemispheres work together. The ancestral images and memories we have about birth come through in our mandala, and this offers healing.

Ancient Buddhists used mandalas in their meditation practices. The circle is found throughout the Universe. We see it in our round belly, the cervix, the sperm, the egg, the Sun, the Moon, the Earth.

Everyone in the Blessingway ceremony can do a mandala, if they like.

You will need:
Paper
Coloured drawing pens
Pencils
Paints
Coloured chalk
Or crayons

To make a mandala, create a circle, and place a dot in the centre of it.

As the celebrant, ask the people in the medicine wheel a question, such as "what are your thoughts on pregnancy?" or "Birth is an opening. What does that look like?" Ask them to draw from the inside of the circle, and to work their way to the outside.

When everyone's finished, ask if anyone would like to share what they've learned from the experience.

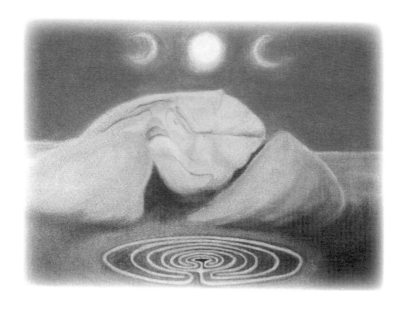

Singing the Songs of the Moon ~ Old Grandmother Turtle, Callanish, by Jill Smith.　　www.jill-smith.co.uk

Labyrinth

A labyrinth is not the same as a maze, but is a single winding path leading to the centre.

Labyrinths have been used for at least 3,500 years, as symbols of our inward journey to our true self, and then back out in the world. They're used not only for deep contemplation, but for centring. In a Blessingway ceremony, you can either do a walking labyrinth (if you have access to a field, beach, large garden or woodland glade) or do a finger-walking labyrinth. Doing either will slow down the brainwaves, and bring balance to mind and body, as well as developing intuition. Pregnancy is a particularly powerful time to use a labyrinth meditation. The inward journey is for letting go or shedding, while the middle of the labyrinth helps us to centre and find stillness. The outward journey is the story of our return and reintegration. The finger labyrinth is particularly useful for a mother who is having a solitary Blessingway ceremony.

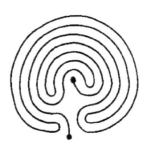

Create your own finger labyrinths.

The nature of labyrinth walking is that it uses the same part of the brain that will be activated in birth. You don't need to be spiritual to take part, however it's beneficial for spiritual growth, as well as for healing, creativity and self-awareness. Tracing a finger labyrinth provides the same sense of a spiritual and meditative journey that many experience in walking an outdoor labyrinth. A finger labyrinth can be made from a patch of fired clay the size of your palm, and then painted. It can also be made from ceramic, lucite, wood, bamboo and pewter. As a celebrant, it's worth keeping one in your medicine bag.

To create a walking labyrinth, you can use candles (inside glass jars), stones, sticks, seashells, driftwood, chalk, dried corn kernels, flour, sawdust, pine cones or other items from Nature.

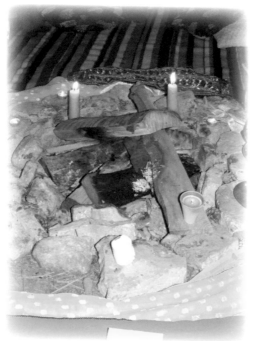

Candles and a small fireplace in the centre of the
roundhouse at the end of a Blessingway ceremony.

The Blessing Candle

Candles are always used in ceremony to represent the fire element, and announce intention as well as to offer light, and at least one should be placed upon the altar. In a Blessingway ceremony, I like to form a circle of candles around the outside of the medicine wheel, where possible. The flame on a candle announces the intention of worship. Colours have special meanings, too. Yellow to symbolise the Sun, white for purity, orange for creativity, green for healing and blue for truth. You can, of course, bring colour into your ceremony in other ways, such as using gemstones, fabric cloths and saris, cushions, lighting.

Please use matches and not a gas lighter when lighting candles in ceremony. Energetically, they feel very different. Don't leave your matches lying on the altar. Place them in a basket or under a cloth.

Choose a beeswax candle (or plant-based one if the mother is a strict vegan). Afterwards, give the candle to the mother so that she can light it when she goes into labour. This will be a beautiful reminder for her of the love, support, wisdom and strength which surrounded her during the Blessingway.

The reason I burn only beeswax candles is because paraffin candles are detrimental to health. Paraffin is a by-product of the petroleum industry. That is, residue from refineries.

Paraffin candles are bleached (which in itself is toxic). Carcinogenic chemicals are used to turn it into a solid product. More chemicals are added, for example: artificial dyes and synthetic fragrances. When these fragrances burn, they release toxic fluorocarbons (and other things), which damage the receptors in your nasal passages. Over time, these sensors lose their ability to detect scent, and you then need stronger-smelling candles or even stronger air fresheners.

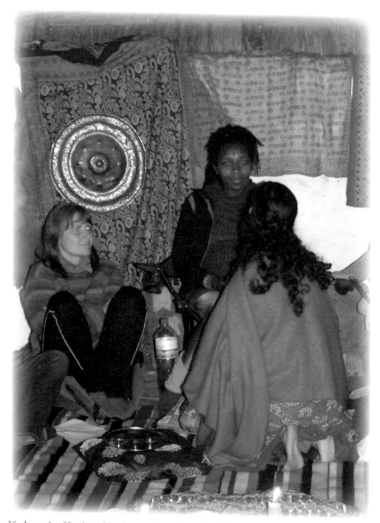

Kalyani offering Vedina a bead and a blessing.

The soot left from paraffin candles coats skin and lungs, as well as household furnishings. Many people, without realising why, suffer from difficulties with their lungs and sinuses, and have allergic reactions and headaches when they burn paraffin.

Like the air after a thunderstorm, beeswax releases negative ions. These attach themselves to positively charged ions (such as airborne contaminants), which then drag them to the ground (to be vacuumed or swept away). Beeswax candles help to clean the air in your home. They burn for much longer than paraffin, so when you're doing a cost comparison, do bear this in mind. Over time, they're far more economical. Make sure that if you're buying beeswax, it contains 100% beeswax, and that the fibre which the wick is made from is also natural. Beeswax candles have a beautiful honey-like scent. If you get scented candles, be sure the essential oils used are 100% pure.

Depending on the number of guests, the mother-to-be might like to give each one a candle to take home and light when they hear news that labour has begun. During the ceremony, they can light their candle from the altar candle for a few moments, before extinguishing it.

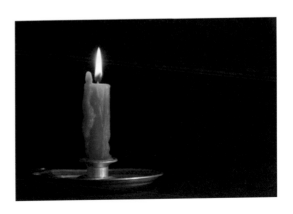

On Children
by Kahlil Gibran

Your children are not your children.
They are the sons and daughters of Life's longing
for itself.
They come through you, but not from you,
and though they are with you yet they belong not to you.

You may give them your love but not your thoughts,
for they have their own thoughts.
You may house their bodies but not their souls,
for their souls dwell in the house of tomorrow,
which you cannot visit, not even in your dreams.

You may strive to be like them,
but seek not to make them like you.
For life goes not backward nor tarries with yesterday.

You are the bows from which your children
as living arrows are sent forth.

The archer sees the mark upon the path of the infinite,
and He bends you with His might
that His arrows may go swift and far.
Let your bending in the archer's hand be for gladness;
for even as He loves the arrow that flies,
so He loves also the bow that is stable.

Word-medicine

"Positive birth stories only, please.
My baby is listening."

Words have power. They can act as swords or as feathers. They have the power to destroy, and the power to heal. In Blessingway, we seek to bring word-medicine through readings, prayers, stories and poems. If guests have been asked to do a reading, encourage them to think closely about the words they're gifting.

Storytelling has long been used in ceremony for its therapeutic benefits. All good stories have purpose, truth and action at their heart.

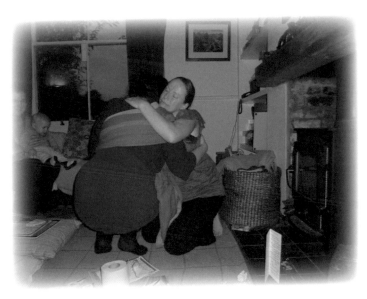

Karen receives kind words during her ceremony.

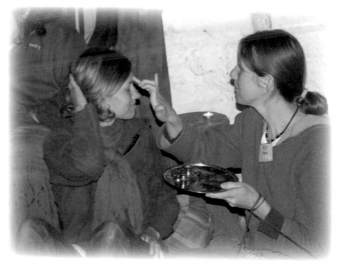

Bindis anointed around the medicine wheel. Above: Jamie and Alex. Below: Alex and Sara.

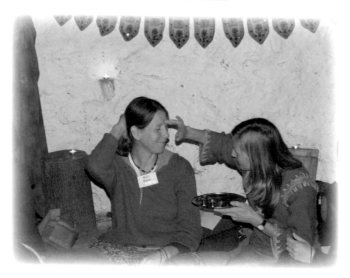

Sound in Ceremony

Music has been used since the dawn of humanity in ritual and worship. Even before the development of language, we would have hummed and made lyrical sounds.

Music and song help to raise the energy in ceremony. You can introduce the sounds of Gregorian music, modern-day Blessingway songs, chanting, singing bowls, bells, flutes, drums, chimes and so on. The mother-to-be ideally chooses the music for her ceremony. As celebrant, you can share with her the many options available, and how they might change or shape a ceremony, and what different sounds and songs will bring to the medicine wheel.

When using Blessingway songs from a CD, it's always nice to find out who the confident singers in a group are, and contact them ahead of time with the tunes and lyrics. This way, their strong voices can lead the group. It's helpful to print lyrics for everyone so they can join in.

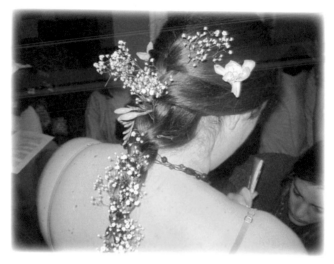

Above: Hair braided with flowers and ribbon.
Below: An ivy crown.

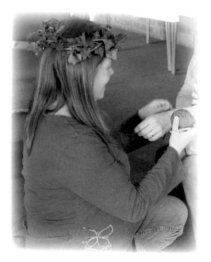

Floral Crown

The Navajo women wear their hair in whorls, but when they prepare to become a mother through the Blessingway ceremony, they tie their hair in a chignon.

In their tradition, it is the mother of the pregnant woman who will comb her hair and change the style during the ceremony, but this role can be taken on by a sister, grandmother or very close friend if the mother isn't available. When the mother brushes her daughter's hair, it evokes memories of a childhood when she often brushed it. Now she'll become a grandmother. This is her journey, too, and she's sharing a ritual across the generations.

In our culture, we tend to change our hair all the time, so we need to seek a way to make this ritual more meaningful. Creating a floral crown satisfies this need.

Each guest will be asked to bring flowers or leaves which can be wound into a grapevine or willow wreath around the mother-to-be's head. If she's not comfortable with this, then stick with braiding her hair and lacing it with ribbon and flowers. Depending on the season, you can use leaves, rosehips, acorns and so on to create a seasonal hair wreath.

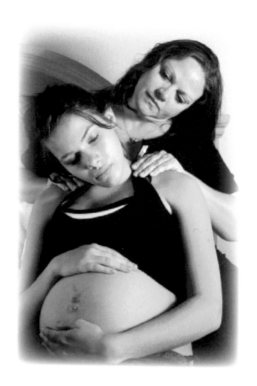

Gentle Touch

One of our most essential needs as human beings is to touch and to be touched, and yet in our modern culture so few of us are regularly held or nurtured in this way. If the mother-to-be is open to it, a Blessingway massage is a beautiful way to honour her. She may prefer a face massage to a belly one, or indeed may prefer to have her feet massaged. If there's a reflexologist in the group, offer this as a gift.

Be mindful of the oils which are used, whether it's the carrier oil or the essential oils. My preferred oils for massage are: unbleached, edible coconut (it may need to be warmed in cooler weather as it's solid below 25C), almond, apricot kernel and grapeseed. Women with nut allergies are often fine with coconut, but always check first. Ensure the essential oils are 100% pure, and not perfumed fragrances.

Keep the rest of her body warm with blankets and shawls. If she's comfortable, add a couple of drops of essential oils: orange, jasmine, lavender.

Jasmine and geranium are good for lifting the mood in the early weeks after birth.

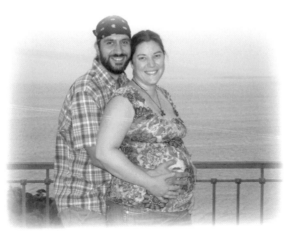

Herbal Foot Bath

Where possible in a Blessingway, use only flowers and herbs which have naturally fallen to the ground. Remembering the symbolism and energy we're trying to create with a Blessingway, we don't want to pick, pull or pluck the plants in a way that is reminiscent of a baby being picked, pulled or plucked at birth (c-section, forceps, ventouse).

Always be mindful of detail, and the power of symbols. Depending on who the guests are at a Blessingway, the ritual herbal foot-washing is often done by the midwife or doula. The ancient tradition of the midwife washing the feet reminds us that her role is a humble one. She is at the feet of the mother.

Traditionally, cornmeal is used to dry the mother's feet. It is rubbed in, and as a form of reflexology opens the woman up for birth. It's also considered an offering from the Corn Mother.

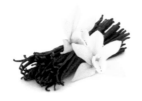

When the belly is well oiled, then begin to add the strips of plaster. Each piece needs to be placed in the warm water, and completely wet. Pull it out of the water gently, and make sure it doesn't curl. Use your fingers to straighten. Let the water drip out, then place a strip over the mother's oiled skin. Use your fingers to smooth it down. Use all the strips until her entire belly (breasts/thighs) is covered.

As part of the drying process, the plaster will pull away from her skin. When you've completed the casting, it will slide off her belly. Take care as you pull it away, and keep it supported while it's drying, which takes about a week. Once it has dried, then it can be decorated.

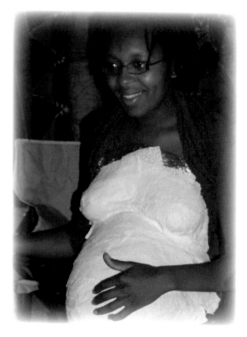

Vedina waiting for the cast to dry.

Mehndi

Henna art can be abstract, or based on Nature, heritage, flowers, leaves, animals, fairies, the celestial, seasons, murals or mosaics.

It's wise to do an allergy check before the ceremony to make sure the mother-to-be isn't sensitive to henna on her skin.

Henna is a tattoo-type artwork which is temporary and washes off within about seven days. The staining is known as *mehndi*. This isn't just about artwork, but has a tradition of protecting the unborn child and the mother. Henna (*Lawsonia Inermis*) has been used for over 9,000 years, often in places such as India and Morocco, both medicinally and cosmetically. It's a small bush that produces a red dye. The dried leaves are ground into powder, then mixed with coffee, fresh lemon juice and essential lavender oil, then formed into a paste.

Don't use black henna ~ this isn't true henna, but a hair dye which contains para-phenylendiamin.

Contraindications for henna art: anaemia, hyperbilirubinemia, immune conditions and blood disorders.

To make henna paste:

1 cup strong coffee
(reduce by boiling till there's half a cup)
1 T lemon juice (fresh)
½ cup fresh sifted henna (not black henna)
3 drops eucalyptus or lavender oil

Mix well, and allow about two hours to cool. You want it to be runny, but not too thin that you can't work with it.

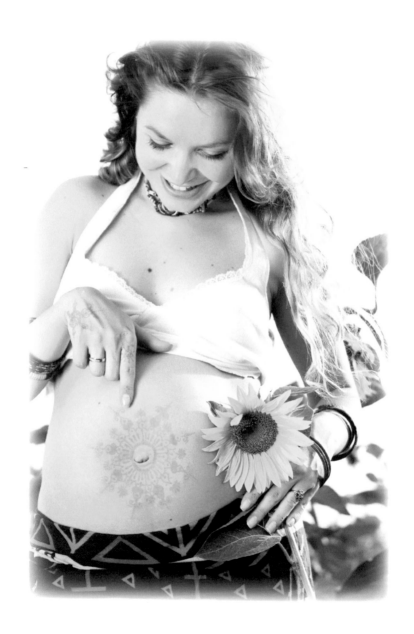

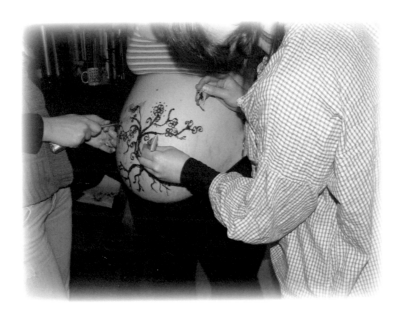

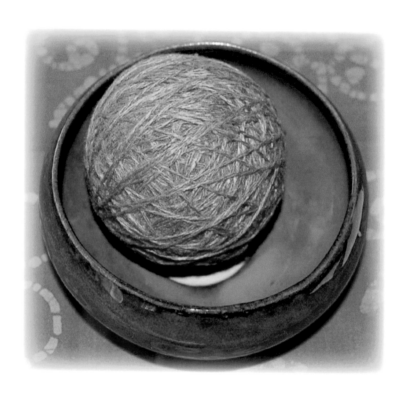

Red Thread

I bring a yarn of red hemp string or wool to the ceremony. This can, of course, be brought by the mother.

I choose red because it's the colour of blood, and is
what links all humans throughout time. During the red-
thread ritual, I pass the ball to the pregnant guest of honour, and she wraps it around her wrist several times, and
then throws the ball across the circle to one of her guests.
That woman also wraps it around her wrist several times
before throwing it to someone else in the circle. This con-
tinues until everyone is linked into the web.

By wrapping the string several times, you'll have
enough to be able to make a braid/plait from it so that
it sits more comfortably around the wrist later on. I like
how the braid becomes 'felted' after being worn for a few
weeks.

As women, we're born from the Earth, and now
we're born into this circle. This is a wonderful symbol of
connection. The guest of honour cuts the string each side
of her wrist, and then cuts the string around the circle.

Each guest wears the string until she hears the joy-
ous news that the baby has been born. (A phone tree is
set up at the end of the ceremony to ensure everyone is
notified.) My Blessingway red-thread braids have gone
on to have new life as bookmarks, and each one always
makes me smile when I think about the woman who had
the ceremony.

As the celebrant, use this weaving time to share
how each of you is united. This bracelet of red thread is
a reminder to offer up conscious prayers for the birthing
mother, and to see her as strong, ecstatic and positive.

Share the story of Tantrika, the Spider Goddess, and
how she weaved the world. As we weave our circle of
sisterhood, we come together all through the One Mother.
Even after the string is cut, we all still come from the same
ball of yarn. Women of the medicine wheel sense this

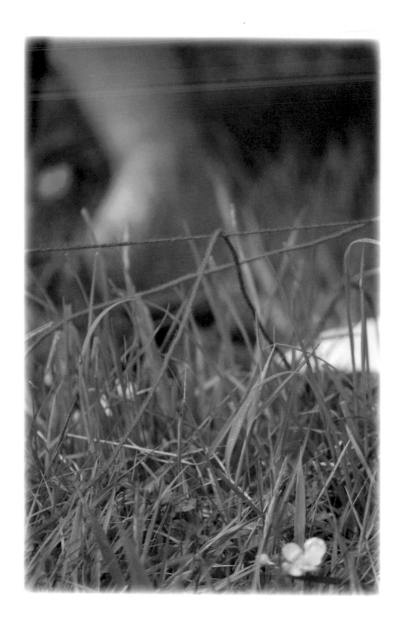

energetically, and really feel connected to the circle in the weeks to come.

In Native American myth, The Spider Grandmother (Spider Woman) created all life by spinning her web, and connected all living life together using her magical thread. The Navajo honoured her. According to myth, she taught people how to weave, as well as other life skills such as planting crops.

The web that is woven in myth also symbolises how we weave a life for ourselves, and have the ability to always choose when to thread next; which way to weave.

We can call to The Spider Grandmother in our day-to-day life when we need guidance about where to weave the next thread of our web.

I wrote about the time I was wearing a red-braided yarn on my wrist after a Blessingway ceremony. It told the story of my life over the next few weeks. Each woman in the medicine circle left with a red thread around her wrist. And in each thread was woven their stories, my story, and every other woman's story. It's a gentle reminder that the love, joy, pain, sadness, exhilaration, fun, torment, inspiration and laughter that fill our body and our life, aren't ours alone ~ they're shared.

If the thread could talk, it would tell you that during those few weeks it witnessed me: weeding the vegetable garden; admiring my sunflowers and the bumblebees and butterflies; bake loaves of sourdough bread; browse a bookshop and find a great CD of music; read Women Who Run With The Wolves; have lovely hugs from my family; snuggle up with my daughters for private chats; enjoy gorgeous support from my friends; receive a phone call from my mum in Tasmania; enjoy Autumnal walks with my family; read inspirational stories; write the book of our family's unschooling journey ~ Life Without School; start healing from months of exhaustion; plant garlic; collect golden sycamore leaves from the village; create a birthing altar; enjoy wild plums; pick pears, apples and courgettes from my garden, and eat fresh sunflower

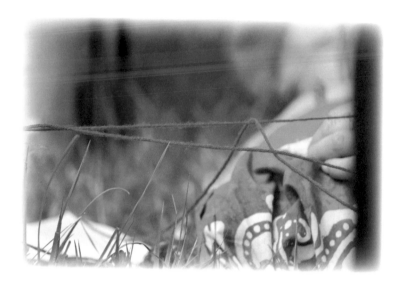

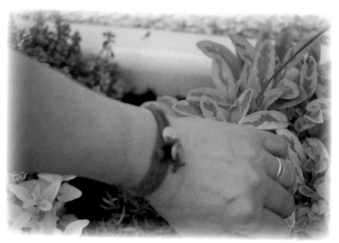

Jacqui wears the red thread as a bracelet.

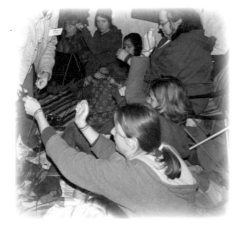

Time to cut the thread.

seeds; and collect starflowers to press in my journal. The thread would tell you that I've had an old friend over for dinner; enjoyed letters and calls from very special friends; listened to the owl last night calling out to me that 'it's time for change'; made ten jars of pickled cucumbers; baked the 'perfect' cake; watched the beautiful stars twinkling in the sky; breathed in beautiful handmade lavender bags which arrived in the post; felt sunshine on my shoulders while going blackberry-picking with my daughter.

Practical tip:
Bring ~ red thread/string/cord/hemp.
Scissors! Forgetting them is not helpful if you're in a remote field and only realise after everyone is tied in the web.

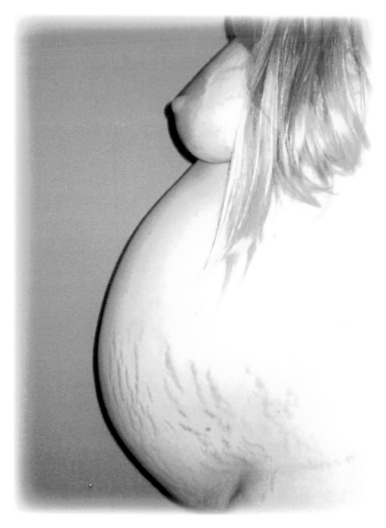

Nature's tattoo ~ beautiful stretch marks.

Gratitude

If the only prayer you say in your life
is 'thank you', that would suffice.
~ Meister Eckhart

For me, a life without gratitude is probably a life not worth living. To be thankful means acknowledging everything you receive, and being aware of the simplest pleasures in life. You see your life as nothing short of a miracle. Gratitude means you live a life of abundance, even if there are only a few pennies in your bank account.

Gratitude centres you, and helps you live in the present moment. It builds your immune system, and leads to happiness.

A celebrant who is grounded in the daily ritual of gratitude brings more to the ceremonies she (he) performs than one who doesn't. It's inherent in her word-medicine, posture and presence.

Gratitude practice:

I start my day by standing at the French doors of my bedroom, and giving thanks for the new day. Even if I don't get to see that big yellow face coming over the horizon because it's shrouded in cloud, I still give thanks.

No matter what someone does for you in the course of a day, learn to say thank you with all your heart.

Make time in your life to write thank-you notes and make thank-you phone calls.

What about the unpleasant things in life? Do we give thanks for them, for the limitations, stresses and challenges? *Yes.* We give thanks that they're on our path, and that we're developing personal growth from the experience. Approaching the negative aspects of life in a creative way can turn them into blessings.

Closing the Circle

The time has come to close the circle. As the celebrant, I acknowledge that the circle will open, but will remain unbroken. Regardless of the circles we create, I always believe the right people will be there and that we have come together for a purpose.

Use this time to express gratitude to those around the medicine wheel, as well as to the ancient mothers and other unseen energies. Thank everyone on behalf of the mother-to-be. The circle may be closed with a song, chant, or quiet prayer. I encourage the participants to hold hands for a moment while still in circle, then I let them know when to let go.

I believe it's important (unless there's an emergency) for everyone who has come for the ceremony to stay there until the circle has closed, as it changes the energy for those left behind.

Song: *Sisters you give me courage*

Sisters you give me courage to carry on,
To open to the strength I know inside.
You help me unlock the love in my heart,
And I am grateful.
© Blessingway Songs CD, Copperwoman

A Solitary Blessingway

If you've read this book and would love a Blessingway, but you've got no close friends or family where you live, what can you do? Create a solitary Blessingway. Obviously there'll be some activities that you can't do on your own, but there are still many ways to conduct a ceremony for yourself that are rich, deep and meaningful. Use the ideas in this book and modify them for your situation. You could invite friends and family from around the world to send you a bead for your birthing necklace, including their wishes for your birth. You can thread this during labour. Make your own prayer flags or ask friends at a distance to make you one; do a finger labyrinth; create a floral crown, and massage your feet after a herbal footbath. You can gift close friends with a candle to light during your labour. As with any ceremony, the intention is what makes it sacred and powerful.

Adoption

Is there any reason that a couple about to adopt a child or children can't have a Blessingway ceremony? Not at all. The essential energy and intention of Blessing the Way can easily be tailor-made to their situation. If you know the names of the children, include them in the ceremony. A man and woman going through the adoption process still need a circle to surround them, sisters (and brothers) to support their journey, and ancient mothers to guide them. They may not have a bellycast made or belly painted, but they most certainly can take part in a labyrinth, make a mandala, enjoy a footbath and have prayer flags, beads and webbing for their parenting journey.

As a celebrant, spend time talking to them about their hopes and fears, and transform this into a positive, life-affirming ceremony.

Timing the Ceremony

It's important when sending out Blessingway invitations to give guests an approximate idea of how long the ceremony will be. Ask them to arrive at least ten minutes before the starting time, and to allow plenty of time for their journey to the venue. As a celebrant, don't start until you know everyone has arrived.

You will have worked with the mother-to-be to decide which elements she'd like included in her ceremony, and you can use these to get an idea of the duration. Also, bear in mind that human emotion needs to be allowed for during the times when guests are sharing.

Opening ceremony = 10 minutes
Footbath = 15 minutes
Hairbrushing = 10 minutes
Floral crown = 10 minutes
Henna = 30 minutes
Body art = 30 minutes
Reflexology = 20 minutes
Massage = 15 minutes
Labyrinth = 30 minutes
Mandala = 30 minutes
Prayer flags = 30 minutes
Blessing box = 15 minutes
Bellycast = 40-50 minutes
Birthing beads = 30 minutes (depending on number of guests)
Red-thread web weaving = 10 minutes
Songs = 20 minutes
Food = 30 minutes
Closing = 5 minutes

Mother Food

Food has bonded and grounded humans throughout time. It activates all the senses, and is a powerful component of ceremonial ritual. Encourage guests to bring a plate of nourishing food to share. I recommend leaving the food until after the ceremonial circle has closed, as it can be too distracting to the intention of the other rituals.

The food could follow a red theme like the red thread, or food specific to the mother's background or heritage. Always ensure that there's food suitable for those with allergies/sensitivities. During the feasting at the end of the Blessingway ceremony, see that the names and phone numbers of each person present are put onto a phone tree (to be used when the baby is born), and for each person to bring a meal after birth. Depending on each person's circumstances, they might offer to come in and help with a job each day such as hanging up the washing, sweeping the floor, watering plants, taking a toddler for a walk, or reading him some stories. This isn't a time for sitting around chatting to mum (she's on a Ba-

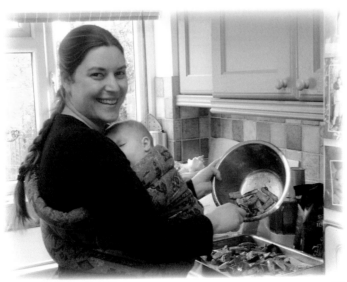

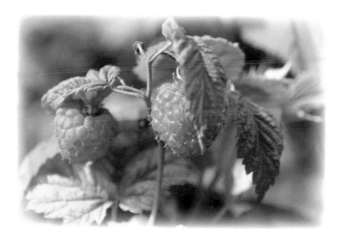

bymoon), but for quietly coming in to help with jobs and then disappearing.

Ensure that food is friendly to the family. For example, check if they're vegan, vegetarian, gluten- or dairy-free, have allergies, and whether they prefer wholefoods; spicy or bland foods, etc., and make sure the foods are breastfeeding-friendly.

Labour candle: While numbers for the phone tree are being collected, the mother-to-be might like one set up for announcing labour has begun, so the guests can light a candle which burns for the duration of her birthing time. This works particularly well if, during the ceremony, she has gifted them candles to light from her birth candle.

Red foods: Cherries, plums, red pears, redcurrants, cranberries, rosehip tea, radishes, tomatoes, tomarillos, red onions, fresh figs, pomegranates, rhubarb, red kidney beans, red peppers, watermelon, strawberries, raspberries, red apples, red rice, red quinoa. So, how about a fruit platter, followed by roast red-pepper soup, sundried tomato and olive bread, salsa, kidney-bean dip? Or strawberry ice cream using fresh strawberries, honey/maple syrup and coconut cream? Maybe a vegan jelly (use agar agar) with strawberries or raspberries.

Invitation

Send invitations out one lunar month (four weeks) before the date of the ceremony. Plan to have the Blessingway at the eighth month of pregnancy, where possible.

You are invited to
join
Seraphina
for her Blessingway ceremony
in honour of the new life she is creating.

2-4pm, Saturday, October 10th.
In the cherry woodland behind Seraphina's house.

Please bring with you a bead for the birthing necklace (made from wood, fabric, glass or other natural product); a naturally fallen flower to weave into the floral crown; a blessing (poem, song, word or sentence); and a small mothering gift for the Blessing box, such as herb tea, plant-based soap, herbs, a beeswax candle.

Please RSVP by October 1st, to Seraphina or (celebrant)
Phone: 897 111

You might like to include a note which explains what a Blessingway is: This isn't a baby shower but a spiritual reflection and celebration as we witness Seraphina on her journey to motherhood. We'll honour and nurture her with shared vegetarian food, our company, Blessingway songs (lyrics attached), red-thread weaving, a beading ceremony and decorating her hair.

This is an important rite of passage in any woman's life, and we wish to mark Seraphina's journey inspired by the roots of the Navajo tradition. Please ask any questions about the ceremony and what might be expected of you.

Sample Ceremony

This is just an outline. You can add, modify and replace according to the needs and desires of the mother.

Begin by ringing the bell three times, and wait for the mother-to-be to enter the circle.

Celebrant: May you be blessed for sharing this special day, and leave all negative thoughts behind you. I'll begin by smudging with sage, during which time we'll enjoy a few moments of silence until I begin talking again. (*Walks around the medicine wheel with sage.*) In the Navajo tradition, let us give thanks to Changing Woman.

I now call in the spirits of the four directions. I call you spirit of the East. I call you spirit of the South. I call you spirit of the West. I call you spirit of the North.
The Blessingway ceremony is as old as the Navajo Indians, and as young as the baby here in utero. Today we affirm Seraphina is to have a beautiful, ecstatic birth experience. That is our wish. Women are sacred, they are goddesses. They are the Mother Earth made manifest. Let the Divine Mother be made manifest in this Blessingway.

Casting the circle
Celebrant: We meet in this sacred space to witness Seraphina on her journey again into motherhood. We call upon our mothers, grandmothers and great-grandmothers throughout time to be with us during this sacred ceremony. We celebrate the long line of women who gave birth to us. I now invite you to join in a Blessingway song.
Song: Circle Surrounding

Celebrant: This candle is to symbolically call in the ancient mothers. (Light candle on altar)

Celebrant: We will now call in the ancient mothers. I will begin, and then ask each of you (*starting with the person on my left*) to introduce yourselves in the same way.

My name is Veronika, and I'm the daughter of Angelikah, granddaughter of Liselotte and Minna Marie.
(*All women in the circle are to introduce themselves this way.*)
Let us now join in song.

Song: Ancient Mother

Beads and blessing
Celebrant: Birth is a spiritual vision quest. It unites the mother-to-be with all women in her chosen community. The beads we gift Seraphina with today are part of a long strand which connects all mothers across time. They bring light to our birthing journey.

As you come up to Seraphina and place your bead in her hands, please state your wish for her birth.
We can now join in song.

Song: Deep down
I am woman deep down (x three)
Oh so deep down.
Verses:
I can love (from deep down)
I can breathe (from deep down)
I open (from deep down)
I give birth (from deep down)
© The Blessingway Songs CD, Copperwoman

Positive Birth stories
Celebrant: This is a time to share positive birth stories with Seraphina. Let us all remember that her baby is listening, too, so may the words you speak be empowering and inspiring.

Henna Art
Celebrant: The staining of henna art is known as mehndi.
It comes from the tradition of protecting the unborn child
and the mother, and as we do this today, we're part of a
line which has used this for over 9,000 years. While this
is being created, you might like to join in a Blessingway
song.

Song: Mama Ocean
Mama, mama ocean
Hold me while I rock and roll in your waves
Mama, mama ocean
Hold me close, tell me your ways.

1. Caress me with that tender touch
I love so much (x 2)

2. I feel your breath inside of me
I surrender, and I am set free (x 2)

3. Tell me the secrets of your deep dark floor
Help me find what I am looking for (x 2)

4. Wave after wave comes tumbling down
Wheel of life turns round and round (x 2)
©The Blessingway Songs CD, Copperwoman

Weaving the thread
Celebrant: We now come to the red-thread ritual. All
women are connected. We once lived in our mother's
watery womb. As an unfertilised egg, you lived in your
grandmother's womb. Motherhood is written within each
one of us, regardless of whether we are mothers, daughters, sisters or friends, and this is true even if we don't
ever give birth ourselves. We are women. We are powerful.

As Seraphina takes the string, she's at the centre of this web of women. As we wrap it around our wrists several times, we will then toss it across the room to another woman, and we'll weave our web. You're invited to wear these as bracelets or anklets until you hear of this baby's arrival Earthside. *(When everyone is part of the web, invite the mother-to-be to cut her string first.)*

Hair braid
Celebrant: Seraphina's mother will now come forward and do the ritual brushing and hairstyle change for Seraphina. While we're witnessing this, you might like to join in the song, Older, Wiser.

Older, wiser, stronger, lighter
As the Winters and the Summers pass us by.
© The Blessingway Songs CD, Copperwoman

Close the circle
Celebrant: We thank our ancient mothers and other unseen guests for joining with us this day. Thank you everyone for coming. You've given with your hearts, minds and company. Thank you. Seraphina and I hope you've received as many blessings this day as she has. May this circle be open, but unbroken. Go in peace. We will now join together for supper.

***

Food ritual: Celebrant to offer grace. For example:

> *Earth who gives us this food*
> *Sun who makes it ripe and good*
> *Dear Earth, dear Sun*
> *By you we live*
> *Our loving thanks to you we give.*

Collate the phone tree for labour and/or postnatal meals and housekeeping support.

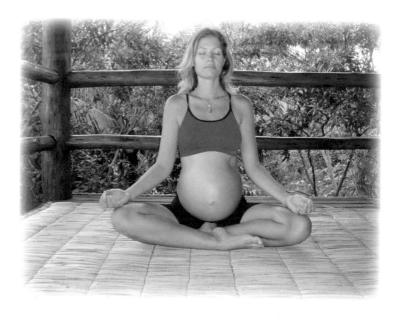

Practising yoga during pregnancy is one way to heal the split between soul and spirit found in our culture. Prenatal yoga sexualises spirituality and spiritualises fertility It is the tantric practice of mothers. Once the babies come planetside, our yoga practice shifts into karma yoga, beyond belief. We become servants to our babies, and our path is bhakti yoga, the practice of devotion. Giving conscious birth is woman's vision quest, par excellence. It is ultimate sadhana, spiritual practice ~ which requires purity in strength, flexibility, health, concentration, surrender, and faith.

~ *Jeannine Parvati Baker*. Prenatal Yoga & Natural Childbirth (2001)

Acknowledgements & Resources

Acknowledgements

With gratitude to Copperwoman for permission to reprint lyrics from the Blessingway Songs CD.
www.copperwoman.com www.blessingwaysongs.org

Photography and artwork
With gratitude to the following people:

Jill Smith for her labyrinth painting: Singing the Songs of the Moon ~ Old Grandmother Turtle, Callanish www.jill-smith.co.uk page 60.

Lorena Leonardis Schernberg for her mandala, *Florecer*. www.SaludArte.ch, www.facebook.com/LoresMandalas page 58.

Photographs:
Kathryn Los, pp. 30, 36, 44, 84, 89, 73, 77
Keeley Farrington, pp. 49, 52, 70, 78.
Jacqui Ferguson, pp. 24, 34, 68, 80, 82.
Karen Tye-Walker, pp. 27, 50, 67.
Jamie Abrams, pp. 19, 20, 31, 32, 55, 56, 96
Cover photo from Istock.

Resources

Blessingway Songs CD by Copperwoman
http://www.copperwoman.com/pages/music.html
www.blessingwaysongs.org

Jewellery
Wild Mother Arts
http://www.wildmotherarts.com/
For an assortment of delightful jewellery, including labyrinth bracelets and earrings.

Red hemp thread
http://hemphutt.com/coloredhemp.html

Candles

http://www.stevalcandlecompany.co.uk/
http://www.beeswaxco.com/
http://www.queenb.com.au/

Mandala prints to purchase for the altar

www.SaludArte.ch, www.facebook.com/LoresMandalas
http://themandalajourney.com/store/prints/

Finger labyrinths and more

www.ispiritual.com/
www.fingerlabyrinths.com/
www.madmoonarts.com
www.sevenstonespottery.com

Books

The Mystic Cookfire: the sacred art of creating food for friends and family, by Veronika Sophia Robinson. More than 260 recipes which can be used to make meals for the new family or for bringing to a Blessingway feast.

The Birthkeepers: reclaiming an ancient tradition, by Veronika Sophia Robinson. A great gift for an expectant mother to re-frame the cultural messages about birth.

References
Blessingway by Leland C. Wyman, 1970, Leland C. Wyman, University of Arizona Press

Navajo Blessingway Singer, the Autobiography of Frank Mitchell, 1881-1967, edited by Charlotte J. Frisbie and David P. McAllester, 1978, University of Arizona Press

About the Author

Veronika Sophia Robinson has been a celebrant since 1995, when she began officiating wedding ceremonies in New Zealand. She has also been a celebrant for the following ceremonies: house blessing; divorce; menarche; menopause; baby naming; Handfasting; Blessingway; letting go; Phoenix. She has officiated ceremonies internationally, in a variety of locations including: Maori marae, botanical gardens, by an ancient spring, bushland, a stone circle, river, fields, Ironage replica roundhouse, yurts and homes.

She was born and raised in South East Queensland, Australia, the fourth of eight children, and enjoyed living in the great Australian bush amongst the eucalyptus trees, red soil, continuous sunshine and kangaroos.

In 1995, she co-founded the National Waterbirth Trust (New Zealand), and in 2002 launched The Mother magazine, to an international readership, from her home in the UK. Alongside editing this unique publication on optimal parenting, her other passions include being a wife and mother, metaphysics and spirituality, psychological astrology, walking, vegetarian cooking, organic gardening by the Moon, living in accord with Nature, yin yoga, self-sufficiency, writing and music.

Veronika lives in a 300-year-old sandstone cottage overlooking fields and fells, with her husband Paul, and their two home-educated daughters, in rural Cumbria in the north of England. Veronika and Paul co-edit and publish The Mother magazine. www.themothermagazine.co.uk (www.themothermagazine.org, for USA and Canada subscriptions). She's available for ceremonies in the north of England and southeast Scotland: http://www.themothermagazine.co.uk/ceremonies/ For mentoring on any aspect of natural parenting and holistic living: www.veronikarobinson.com or visit The Mother website for an astrological consultation.

About The Mother Magazine

The Mother magazine was conceived in late 2001, and in February 2002 the first issue was published. Each issue of The Mother is gestated and birthed within the walls of their old cottage at the base of the North Pennines, in rural Cumbria, England.

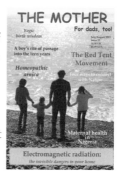

Articles are edited, photos and illustrations chosen, and pages are laid out against the backdrop of family life: soup simmering on the stove, cats sleeping on the sofa, a daughter playing the violin, or another writing a novel by the woodstove. The essence of this grass-roots approach to a professional publication is to bring heart and soul to the families around the world who read The Mother.

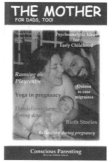

The purpose of this publication isn't to prescribe a way of parenting, but to help women and men access their deep, intuitive knowing, and find a way to parent optimally. The Mother covers many topics and aspects of natural family living, from conscious conception and fertility awareness, to organic birth and death, peaceful pregnancy, human-scale education, natural beauty and cleaning products and toys, vaccine awareness and natural immunity, teenagers, rites of passage, electromagnetic radiation, Moontime, full-term breastfeeding, the family bed and attachment parenting.

We recognise that modern technology is here to stay, and we aim to inform readers about how this can impact on a child's well-being and development.

At times, most of us compromise the optimal, both in terms of parenting, and life in general. We encourage taking responsibility for the outcomes of our choices, actions and inaction. If you've enjoyed reading The Blessingway, then we invite you to join The Mother magazine's family.
www.themothermagazine.co.uk or
www.themothermagazine.org (for USA and Canada.)

About Starflower Press

Starflower Press is dedicated to publishing material which lifts the heart, and helps to raise human consciousness to a new level of awareness.

It draws its name and inspiration from the olden-day herb, Borage (Borago Officinalis), commonly known as Starflower, which is still found in many places, though it's often thought of as a wild flower, rather than a herb.

Starflower is recognisable by its beautiful star-like flowers, which are formed by five petals of intense blue (sometimes it's pink). The unusual blue colour was used in Renaissance paintings. The Biblical meaning of this blue is *heavenly grace*.

Borage, from the Celt borrach, means *courage*. Throughout history, Starflower has been associated with courage. It is used as a food, tea, tincture and flower essence to bring joy to the heart and gladden the mind.

Visit www.starflowerpress.com

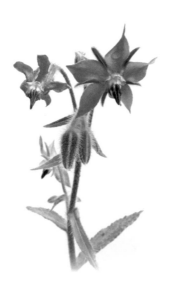

From the heart of Earth, by means of yellow pollen
Blessing is extended.
Blessing is extended.
On top of a pollen floor may I there in blessing give birth!
With long life-happiness surrounding me
May I in blessing give birth!
May I quickly give birth!
In blessing may I arise again, in blessing may I recover,
As one who is long life-happiness may I live on!

-Navajo chant from the Blessingway Ceremony

Blessingway notes

Lightning Source UK Ltd.
Milton Keynes UK
UKRC01n1841130917
309140UK00001B/1

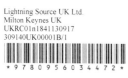